Copyright 2023

All right reserved.No part of this book should be reproduced without express permission of the author.

Reproduction of all or any part of this book is punishable unders relevant law.

Table of Contents

PREVIEW

Autism spectrum disorders (ASD) are a diverse group of conditions. They are characterised by some degree of difficulty with social interaction and communication. Other characteristics are atypical patterns of activities and behaviours, such as difficulty with transition from one activity to another, a focus on details and unusual reactions to sensations.

The abilities and needs of autistic people vary and can evolve over time. While some people with autism can live independently, others have severe disabilities and require life-long care and support. Autism often has an impact on education and employment opportunities. In addition, the demands on families providing care and support can be significant. Societal attitudes and the level of support provided by local and national authorities are important factors determining the quality of life of people with autism.

Characteristics of autism may be detected in early childhood, but autism is often not diagnosed until much later.

People with autism often have co-occurring conditions, including epilepsy, depression, anxiety and attention deficit hyperactivity disorder as well as challenging behaviours such as difficulty sleeping and self-injury. The level of intellectual functioning among autistic people varies widely, extending from profound impairment to superior levels.

AUTISM DIET RECIPES

BREAKFAST

1. Baked Chorizo & Eggs with Peperonata

Prep Time: 10 Minutes

Cook Time: 1hrs 5 Minutes

Servings: 6

Ingredients

Peperonata

- 4 tbsp (60 ml) olive oil
- 4 red, yellow or orange bell peppers, deseeded and sliced
- 1 red onion, finely sliced
- 2 garlic cloves, minced
- 6 plum tomatoes, quartered, deseeded and sliced
- 1 tbsp sugar
- 3 tbsp (45 ml) balsamic vinegar
- Freshly ground black pepper

- Eggs & Chorizo
- 1/2lb (250g) cooking chorizo sausages, peeled and cut into 2cm cubes
- 1 large handful fresh parsley, chopped
- 6 large eggs
- 1/4 cup (25 g) grated parmesan (omit or replace with dairy free parmesan if needed)
- freshly ground black pepper

Instructions

Peperonata

1. Warm the oil in a large oven-safe pan or skillet over a medium heat. Add the peppers, onion and garlic and cook 15 minutes, stirring every so often to keep things from burning.
2. Add the tomatoes, sugar and balsamic vinegar. Mix and cook another 20 minutes over a medium-low heat until the mixture transforms into a chunky sauce-like consistency. Stir every so often.
3. Chorizo & Egg Bake
4. Preheat oven to 350°F/180°C.
5. Heat another medium-sized pan over a medium high heat. Add the diced chorizo and fry for about 4-5

minutes until crispy edges form. Remove from the heat until the peperonata is done.

6. Add the chorizo and half the parsley to the peperonata mixing everything together thoroughly. Using the back of a spoon, spread the mixture evenly across the skillet then make six small holes (for the eggs) across the mixture.

7. Carefully crack the eggs into the little holes. Sprinkle the parmesan over the top and place in the oven to bake for 12-15 minutes until the eggs have cooked but are still a little runny.

8. Sprinkle over the remaining parsley and freshly ground black pepper over the top and enjoy.

Prep Time: 15 Minutes

Cook Time: 30 Minutes

Servings: 12

Ingredients

- 4 eggs
- 1 teaspoon (5 ml) vanilla extract
- 1/2 cup coconut sugar
- 1/2 cup (104 g) coconut oil, melted & cooled
- 2 mashed ripe bananas , about 1 cup (the darker/spottier the better)
- 1/2 cup (50 g) almond flour (can be subbed with tapioca flour 55 g)
- 1/2 cup (56) coconut flour
- 1 teaspoon baking powder
- 1 teaspoon cinnamon
- 1/4 teaspoon sea salt
- 1/4 cup walnuts, chopped (optional)

Crumb Topping:

- 2 tablespoons almond flour (can be subbed with tapioca flour)
- 2 tablespoons coconut flour
- 1/4 cup coconut sugar
- 1 teaspoon ground cinnamon
- 2 tablespoons coconut oil, melted and cooled
- 2 tablespoons walnuts, chopped

Instructions

1. Preheat your oven to 400°F/200°C. Grease or line a 12 cup muffin tin. Set aside.
2. Beat the eggs in a medium sized bowl. Add the vanilla, sugar and the oil to the eggs, mixing thoroughly. In a separate small bowl mash the bananas removing as many lumps as you can. Stir in the mashed bananas in with the egg mixture.
3. Add the dry ingredients to the bowl: (almond flour flour, coconut flour, baking powder, cinnamon, salt and walnuts) and mix until well combined.
4. Scoop the batter out and into the prepared muffins tins. Fill about 3/4 of the way full.

Crumb Topping

1. Wipe down the bowl you used to make the batter and add the the flours, coconut sugar, cinnamon and walnuts (if using) for the topping. Once combined add in the melted coconut oil. Mix into a crumbly mixture.

2. Sprinkle the crumb mixture over the top of the muffins and gently press the crumb into the top of the batter.

3. Place in the bottom third of the oven and bake for 28-30 minutes or until cooked in the centre. To check for doneness prick the centre of the cake with a knife or toothpick - if it comes out clean it's done.

Prep Time: 15 Minutes

Cook Time: 20 Minutes

Servings: 12

Ingredients

- 1 tbsp (15 ml) olive oil
- 1/2 cup (80 g) yellow onion, sautéed
- 6 eggs
- 1 cup (240 ml) milk or cream
- 1 teaspoon garlic, minced
- 1/2 teaspoon salt
- 1/4 teaspoon cayenne
- 1 cup (113 g) grated cheddar
- 2 cups broccoli florets, chopped fine (about 1 small/medium head)

Instructions

1. Preheat oven to 350°F/180°C. Lightly grease or line a 12 cup muffin tin and set aside.

2. Warm the olive oil in a skillet over a medium heat. When the oil is hot add the onion and sauté for about 4-5 minutes until softened. Add the broccoli and garlic and cook another 2-3 minutes.

3. In a large mixing bowl, whisk together the eggs, milk, salt and cayenne until well mixed. Stir in the cheese.

4. Evenly divide the chopped broccoli pieces and sautéed onion between muffin cups.

5. Pour the egg mixture over the broccoli. Fill the cups up about 3/4 of the way full. Place in the middle of the preheated oven and bake uncovered for 20-22 minutes or until the tops are firm the eggs are no longer jiggly.

6. Let the muffins cool for about 10 minutes in the pan before removing. Run a knife around the edges of the muffins to help release the muffins from the pan.

Prep Time: 15 Minutes

Cook Time: 20 Minutes

Servings: 12

Ingredients

- 1 egg wrap
- 1 teaspoon olive oil
- 1 big handful spinach
- 1 tablespoon cream cheese
- 2 sun dried tomatoes in oil, blot the oil and dice
- 1/4 teaspoon dried oregano
- pinch of salt + pepper
- 1 ounce feta, crumbled

Instructions

1. Warm the olive oil in a small pan and add the spinach. Cook for 1-2 minutes until the spinach has darkened and wilted and then remove from heat.

2. Add the spinach to a small bowl along with the cream cheese, sun dried tomatoes, oregano, salt and pepper. Mix everything together and taste to season if needed.

3. Lay the prepared egg wrap out on a flat surface. Spread the cream cheese mixture across the surface and sprinkle the feta over the top.

4. Roll the wrap to close. You can enjoy as is or wrap up to save for later. To warm up the filling: secure the ends of the wrap with a couple of toothpicks and then place on a small/medium skillet over a medium low heat. Cook each side for 30-60 seconds to warm through and enjoy.

5. These wraps can keep up to 2 days.

Prep Time: 15 Minutes

Cook Time: 40 Minutes

Servings: 8

Ingredients

- 4 large bell peppers, cut in half lengthwise and remove inner seeds and stems
- 1 tablespoon olive oil
- 1 cup white onion
- 1 pound gluten free pork sausage, casing removed
- 2 cups spinach
- 4 large eggs
- 1/4 teaspoon salt & pepper, each
- 3/4 cup shredded mozzarella

Instructions

1. Preheat oven to 350°F/180°C. Lightly grease a 9x13 baking dish.
2. Arrange the bell peppers side-by-side in the greased baking dish - cut side up. Set aside

Filling

1. Warm the olive oil to a large skillet over a medium heat. Add the onions and cook about 5 minutes to soften. Add the sausage and cook until no longer pink. Stir in the spinach and cook an addition 1-2 minutes until wilted. Remove from the heat.
2. In a medium sized mixing bowl whisk together the eggs, salt and pepper. Stir in 1/2 cup of the cheese.

Assembly

1. Spoon the sausage mixture evenly into your prepared peppers. Pour the egg mixture over the top of the sausage. Top with the remaining 1/4 cup cheese.
2. Return to the oven and bake an additional 35-40 minutes until the cheese has goldened.

Prep Time: 15 Minutes

Cook Time: 20 Minutes

Servings: 8

Ingredients

- 2 tablespoons butter, dairy free if needed
- 1/3 cup rice flour
- 1/3 cup tapioca flour or corn starch
- 1/4 teaspoon salt
- 2 whole eggs
- 1/2 cup milk, any type of milk will work - non dairy if needed)
- 1 teaspoon vanilla extract
- Optional Toppings
- sprinkle of powdered sugar
- maple syrup or honey
- fresh fruit

Instructions

1. Preheat oven to 220°C/425°F. Add the butter to a 10 inch cast iron skillet or oven dish and place in the oven as it heats up.

2. In a medium sized mixing bowl whisk together the flours and salt.

3. Add the eggs and mix well until no lumps remain. You should have a very thick, smooth batter at this point.

4. Stir in the milk and vanilla until you have a thin batter.

5. After the oven has fully heated and the butter has melted remove the skillet/baking dish from the oven. Swirl the dish around so that the melted butter coats the bottoms and sides.

6. Pour the batter in the skillet/dish and place back in the oven on a middle rack. Let cook 20-22 minutes until puffed and lightly browned on top. Add your toppings if any and enjoy warm.

Prep Time: 15 Minutes

Cook Time: 20 Minutes

Servings: 12

Ingredients

- 4 eggs
- 1 teaspoon (5 ml) vanilla extract
- 1/4 cup (85 g) honey, or maple syrup (use maple for low FODMAP)
- 1/2 cup (104 g) coconut oil, melted & cooled
- 2 mashed ripe bananas , about 1 cup (the darker/spottier the better)
- 1/2 cup (55 g) tapioca flour
- 1/2 cup (56) coconut flour
- 1 teaspoon baking soda
- 1 teaspoon cinnamon
- 1/4 teaspoon sea salt
- 1/3 cup (57 g) dairy free, paleo friendly chocolate chips

Instructions

1. Preheat your oven to 350°F/180°C. Grease or line a 12 cup muffin tin. Set aside.

2. Beat the eggs in a medium sized bowl. Add the vanilla, honey (or maple) and the oil to the eggs, mixing thoroughly. In a separate small bowl mash the bananas removing as many lumps as you can. Stir in the mashed bananas in with the egg mixture.

3. Add the dry ingredients to the bowl: (tapioca flour, coconut flour, baking soda, cinnamon and salt) and mix until well combined.

4. Stir in the chocolate chips. Optional: save a few chocolate chips to sprinkle over the top of the muffin batter just before baking.

5. Scoop the batter out and into the prepared muffins tins. Fill about 3/4 of the way full. Drop a few extra chocolate chips over the batter and bake in the middle of the oven.

6. Bake for 18-20 minutes. To check for doneness - insert a toothpick or a knife in the centre of any muffin. If it comes out clean without any crumbs they're done.

7. Let muffins cool for about 10 minutes before removing and enjoy!

Prep Time: 15 Minutes

Cook Time: 25 Minutes

Servings: 6

Ingredients

- 1 3/4 cup | 220g gluten free all purpose flour blend
- 1 1/4 teaspoon xanthan gum
- 1/2 cup | 100g coconut sugar or light brown sugar
- 1 tablespoon baking powder
- 1/4 teaspoon salt
- 1 1/2 teaspoon pumpkin spice (or just use more cinnamon if you want), see notes
- 1 teaspoon ground cinnamon
- 1/4 cup | 55 g coconut oil (creamy and somewhat solid - not melted or in a liquid state)
- 1/2 cup | 112 g coconut milk, full fat & from a can
- 1/2 cup pumpkin puree
- course turbinado or cane sugar, optional for sprinkling on top of the scones

Maple Glaze:

- 1/2 cup | 56g sifted powdered sugar
- 1-2 tablespoons | 15-30 ml maple syrup
- 1/2 teaspoon pumpkin spice

Instructions

1. Whisk together the flour, xanthan, sugar, baking powder, salt and pumpkin spice together in a large mixing bowl and combine.
2. Add the coconut oil to the flour and use a fork to mix into the flour. Mix until the coconut oil is well combined. Your mixture should be powdery & dry.
3. Add the coconut milk and pumpkin to the bowl and stir until a soft dough forms.
4. Turn the dough out onto a sheet of lightly floured parchment paper. Mould the dough into a round disk, about 7 inches wide and 1 1/2 -2 inches tall. Cut the dough into 6 wedges.
5. Place the dough in the fridge for at least 20 minutes. Don't skip this step - the coconut oil needs to harden up so the scones don't spread too much while baking.
6. Preheat the oven to 400°F/200°C. When you're ready to bake transfer the dough to a baking sheet, pull the wedges apart leaving space between each wedge (at

least 2 inches). Sprinkle with course sugar if using and bake for 20-22 minutes until the scones have risen and are golden in colour.

Maple Glaze

1. Mix together the powdered sugar and maple syrup in a small bowl until you get a thick glaze. Start with 1 tablespoon of maple and add an additional tablespoon if you need a more fluid glaze. Drizzle the glaze over the top when the scones are still a little warm and enjoy!

Prep Time: 10 Minutes

Cook Time: 15 Minutes

Servings: 14

Ingredients

- 1 tablespoons | 15 ml coconut oil
- 2 cups |160 grams large unsweetened coconut flakes
- 1/4 cup | 35 grams sunflower seeds
- 1/4 cup | 25 grams pepitas (hulled pumpkin seeds)
- 2 tablespoons | 20 grams chia seeds
- 1 cup | 170 grams mixed nuts (I used a combo cashews & pecans)
- 1 teaspoon ground turmeric
- 1 teaspoon ground cinnamon
- 1 teaspoons | 5 ml vanilla extract
- 3 tablespoons | 45 ml maple syrup

Instructions

2. In a medium sized mixing bowl mix together the coconut, seeds, nuts, cinnamon and turmeric.

3. In a large non stick skillet, heat the coconut oil on a medium-low heat.

4. Add the nut and seed mixture to the warmed skillet and toast, stirring constantly for 5 minutes. You need to keep stirring to keep from burning.

5. Stir in the vanilla extract and maple and cook for another 3-4 minutes. The mixture will be sticky and starting to turn golden brown. Remove from the heat.

6. Line a large baking sheet with baking paper and transfer the granola to the sheet, spreading out in an even layer to let the granola cool into crunchy clusters.

Prep Time: 20 Minutes

Cook Time: 15 Minutes

Servings: 10

Ingredients

- 2 1/4 cup | 230 grams chickpea flour
- 1 tablespoon baking powder
- 2 teaspoons cinnamon
- 1/4 cup | 55 grams soft coconut oil
- 3 ripe | about 300 grams bananas
- 1/2 cup | 112.5 grams full fat coconut milk
- 1/4 cup | 50 grams coconut sugar
- 1 cup | 125 grams chopped walnuts

Maple Glaze

- 1 cup 110 grams powdered sugar, sifted
- 2 tablespoons 30 ml maple syrup
- 1-2 teaspoons 5-10 ml almond milk (or milk of your choice)

LUNCH

Prep Time: 20 Minutes

Cook Time: 15 Minutes

Servings: 4

Ingredients

Balsamic Vinaigrette

- 1/3 cup extra-virgin olive oil (80 ml)
- 2 tablespoons balsamic vinegar (30 ml)
- 1 teaspoon maple syrup (5 ml)
- 1 small clove garlic, finely minced
- 1/2 teaspoon salt
- 1/4 teaspoon ground black pepper

Salad

- 2 boneless, skinless chicken breasts
- 6 cups mixed salad (I used a blend of spinach, arugula and red cos lettuce)
- 2 cups sliced strawberries (10 oz)

- 1/2 red onion, thinly sliced

- 1 avocado, diced

- 1/4 cup roughly chopped walnuts (29 g)

Instructions

Balsamic Vinaigrette

1. Make the vinaigrette by adding the olive oil, balsamic vinegar, maple syrup, garlic, salt and pepper to a cup or jar and whisk well. Taste and season with additional salt and pepper if needed.

Chicken Prep

2. Cut the chicken in half lengthwise so that you end up with 4 smaller, thin fillets. Sprinkle both sides of the chicken breasts with salt and pepper.

3. Heat a large skillet over a medium-high heat. Add 2 tablespoons of the balsamic vinaigrette to the pan. When the vinaigrette is hot add the chicken pieces and cook about 5-6 minutes until browned. Flip the chicken oven and cook the other side about 3-4 minutes until the chicken is browned and cooked through. The vinaigrette will form a glaze on the chicken that should brown nicely. Make sure to stir

around the chicken every so often to keep from burning.

4. Remove the chicken from the heat and cut into cubes. Set aside as you prep your salad.

Salad Assembly

1. Add the salad mix to a large salad bowl along with the strawberries, onion, avocado and walnuts. Add the chicken. Toss the salad together to mix.
2. Pour the remaining vinaigrette over the salad and toss once more to fully coat everything in the vinaigrette.
3. Season the salad with more black pepper and enjoy.

Prep Time: 10 Minutes

Cook Time: 15 Minutes

Servings: 6

Ingredients

Salad

- 5 strips streaky bacon
- 1 pound brussels sprouts, hard ends trimmed
- 1 large apple, cored and diced
- 1/2 cup almonds, chopped
- Optional Additions: crumbled goats cheese or feta, dried cranberries, handful of other chopped nuts like walnut and pecans

Honey Mustard Vinaigrette

- 3/4 cup (180 ml) extra-virgin olive oil
- 2 tbsp (30 ml) white wine vinegar
- 2 tbsp honey
- 1 tbsp mustard
- 1 small clove garlic, mined

- 1/2 tsp salt or to taste
- Freshly ground black pepper or to taste

Instructions

Prep The Sprouts:

1. Cut off the tough ends of the sprouts and any browning outer leaves. Slice them as through thinly as possible and then roughly chop the sliced spouts to make them even smaller.
2. Alternatively you can do this easily using a food processor by using the slicing blade and pressing the sprouts against the blade with the provided plastic pusher.

Salad

1. Once the sprouts are chopped and sliced place them in fine mesh strainer/colander and rinse with water to clean out the dirt that's usually hiding between their leaves.
2. Lay out the bacon on the cold skillet or pan. Turn the heat on low and let the bacon cook for 2-3 minutes until crispy and brown. Flip it over and continue cooking the other side another 2-3 minutes. Remove

the bacon from the pan and place a cutting board. When the bacon is cool enough to handle chop into small bit sized pieces.

3. Add the brussels sprouts, bacon, apple and almonds to a large salad bowl and toss well to combine.

Vinaigrette

1. Add all of the ingredients listed for the vinaigrette to a small cup or jar and whisk until fully combined. Taste and season with more salt and pepper if needed.

2. Just before serving, pour the vinaigrette over the salad and toss to coat.

Prep Time: 10 Minutes

Cook Time: 25 Minutes

Servings: 8

Ingredients

- 1 tablespoons coconut oil
- 1 medium white onion, chopped
- 3 cloves garlic, crushed
- 1 inch chunk ginger, grated (about 1/2 teaspoon ground)
- 1 tablespoon ground turmeric
- 1 teaspoon ground cumin
- 1 tablespoon curry powder
- 1 cup uncooked quinoa
- 1 can | 14 oz/400 grams crushed tomatoes
- 2 cups vegetable stock
- 1 cup coconut milk from a can (ideally use full fat)
- 1 head cauliflower chopped in bite sized pieces
- 3 cups spinach

Instructions

1. Add the coconut oil to a large skillet or pot and warm on medium high heat. When the oil starts to simmer add the onions, ginger and garlic and sauté until softened, about 5 minutes.

2. Add the ground turmeric, cumin, curry powder, salt and pepper. Stir and fry gently cooking another 2 minutes. Add a splash of water if the pot gets too dry.

3. Add quinoa, tomatoes, vegetable stock, coconut milk and cauliflower. Stir the combine and then bring the mixture to a boil. Let boil about a minute before reducing the temperature down till it's simmering. Cover and let cook 15-20 minutes, stirring every so often to keep the bottom from sticking.

4. Uncover then stir in the spinach until wilted. Top with fresh cilantro and serve.

Prep Time: 20 Minutes

Cook Time: 1hrs 25 Minutes

Servings: 8

Ingredients

Crust:

- 3 cups | 350 grams grated zucchini, about 2 large zucchini - squeeze out as much liquid from the zucchini before adding it to the mix
- 1/4 teaspoon salt and pepper
- 1 egg, whisked

Filling:

- 2 eggs
- 200 grams | 7 ounces feta, crumbled
- 9 cups | 260 grams spinach
- 1 cup cherry tomatoes, cut in half and seeds removed

Instructions

Crust

1. Preheat oven to 400°F/205°C. Lightly grease a 9-inch pie pan. Set aside.

2. In a medium sized bowl mix together the grated zucchini, salt, pepper and egg until combined.

3. Gently press the mix into the prepared pie pan. Press evenly into the bottom and side to form a crust. Bake for 25 minutes or until the crust is set and the sides begin to brown.

Filling

1. Add the spinach to large non stick skillet over a medium heat. Cover and let the spinach wilt, 2-3 minutes. Remove from the heat and let cool a few minutes.

2. Whisk the eggs in a medium sized bowl. Stir in the crumbled feta

3. Mix the spinach into the egg-feta mixture.

4. Pour the filling over the crust - spread so it bakes evenly. Lay the cherry tomatoes over the top of the filling in an evenly layer.

5. Reduce oven temperature to 375°F/190°C. Bake for 30-35 minutes or until the filling is set. Let cool for a few minutes before slicing and serving.

Prep Time: 20 Minutes

Cook Time: 45 Minutes

Servings: 4-6

Ingredients

- Squid:
  500 Grams Frozen Squid Tubes
- ½ Cup Plain Flour
- ½ Cup Semolina Flour
- ⅓ Cup Fine Polenta
- 2 Teaspoons Garlic Powder
- 2 Teaspoons Chipotle Powder
- 1 Teaspoon Table Salt
- Vegetable Oil, For Frying
- 2 Cloves Garlic, Finely Sliced
- 1 Red Chilli, Sliced
- Olive Oil
- Finely Grated Zest ½ Lime, Plus Juice To Serve
- Sea Salt

Instructions

1. Defrost and rinse the squid tubes, then cut into shapes. I like to do a combination of rings and lattice-scored rectangles.

2. In a large bowl, combine the flours, polenta, garlic powder, chipotle powder and salt.

3. Heat 5cm of vegetable oil to 180°C in a large saucepan. Dredge the squid in the flour mixture and fry in batches until golden and crisp. Remove with a slotted spoon and drain on a tray lined with paper towels.

4. In a small frying pan, briefly fry the garlic and chilli in a little olive oil until the garlic is just starting to colour.

5. In a large bowl, toss together the squid, lime zest, fried garlic and chilli and sea salt to taste.

6. Serve hot with mayonnaise and a squeeze of lime juice.

Prep Time: 30 Minutes

Cook Time: 1hrs 45 Minutes

Servings: 3

Ingredients

Spice Mix:

- 2 tablespoons coriander seeds
- 2 tablespoons cumin seeds
- 1 teaspoon white peppercorns
- 1 teaspoon Sichuan peppercorns
- 1 tablespoon salt
- 1 tablespoon sugar
- 1 teaspoon garlic powder
- 3 tablespoons chilli flakes
- ½ teaspoon chilli powder, optional

Skewers:

- 600-800 grams lamb shoulder or leg, with fat
- 1 onion
- 1 tablespoon table salt
- ½ cup rice wine

- 1 teaspoon cracked black pepper
- ¼ teaspoon ground white pepper
- Equipment: 10-12 x 8-10-inch bamboo or metal skewers. If using bamboo skewers, soak in warm water for 1 hour before cooking.

Instructions

1. SPICE MIX:Toast the seeds and peppercorns in a dry pan over a medium heat for about 5 minutes, or until aromatic. In a mortar and pestle or spice grinder, grind the toasted components along with the salt, sugar, garlic powder, chilli flakes and chilli powder, if using, until you have a fine powder. Set aside.
2. SKEWERS:Trim any large surface area of fat off the lamb. Cut the fat into chunks and reserve. Cut the lamb meat into 2-3cm cubes.
3. Blanch the lamb fat in 1 litre of boiling water over a high heat for about 4 minutes, or until solid. Remove the fat from the water and shake off excess liquid. Allow to cool slightly, then cut into 2cm cubes. Discard the blanching liquid.

4. Peel the onion and cut into large chunks. It is only used to impart flavour to the meat. In a large bowl, combine the lamb, lamb fat, onion chunks, salt, rice wine, black pepper and white pepper. Cover and marinate in the fridge for at least 2 hours, or up to overnight.

5. Thread the lamb and fat alternately onto the skewers, so there are 4-5 pieces of meat on each skewer. Discard the onions.

6. Heat a grill pan or barbecue to maximum heat. Grill the skewers for 2-3 minutes on each of the 4 sides. Sprinkle a generous amount of the spice mix over the skewers each time you turn them. You should end up with charred edges on the lamb and crispy, rendered fat.

Prep Time: 20 Minutes

Cook Time: 1hrs 15 Minutes

Servings: 6-8

Ingredients

Salmon:

- 1.5-kilogram (approx) side of salmon
- 2 tablespoons extra-virgin olive oil
- 4 cloves garlic, crushed
- 2 tablespoons pomegranate molasses
- 1 teaspoon cumin seeds
- 1 teaspoon sumac
- 1 teaspoon sea salt

Tahini Yoghurt Mayo:

- 1 cup thick plain yoghurt
- ¼ cup good-quality egg mayonnaise
- ¼ cup tahini
- finely grated zest 1 lemon
- 1 clove garlic, crushed
- 1 teaspoon each ground cumin and sea salt

Pickled Red Onions

- ¼ cup cider vinegar
- 2 teaspoons caster sugar
- ½ teaspoon sea salt
- 1 small red onion, thinly sliced

To Serve

- ⅔ cup chopped walnuts, toasted
- 1/3 cup each fresh coriander and mint leaves
- Equipment: Line an oven tray with baking paper.

Instructions

1. Preheat the oven to 220°C fan bake.

Salmon:

2. Lay the salmon skin side down on the lined oven tray. Combine the olive oil, garlic, pomegranate molasses, cumin seeds, sumac and salt. Brush over the salmon and bake for 12 minutes. Take care to not overcook it.

Tahini Yoghurt Mayo:

3. Whisk all the ingredients together until smooth and creamy.

Pickled Red Onions:

4. Put the vinegar, sugar and salt in a small non-reactive bowl and whisk to dissolve the sugar. Add the onion, cover and refrigerate until ready to use.

To Serve:

5. When ready to serve, garnish the salmon with the drained onion, walnuts and herbs. Serve with the Tahini Yoghurt Mayo.

Prep Time: 20 Minutes

Cook Time: 1hrs 15 Minutes

Servings: 6-8

Ingredients

Spice Paste

- 5 cloves garlic
- 1 tablespoon each ground coriander and cumin
- 1 teaspoon each ground cardamom, allspice and sea salt
- ½ teaspoon ground cayenne pepper
- 2 tablespoons pomegranate molasses
- ¼ cup olive oil
- 1.5-kilogram boneless lamb shoulder

To Cook

- 2 large brown onions, peeled and thickly sliced
- 1½ teaspoons sea salt
- 1 teaspoon cumin seeds

Green Chilli Relish

- 1 cup each parsley, mint and coriander leaves
- 3 cloves garlic, roughly chopped
- finely grated zest 1 lemon
- 3-4 green chillies, roughly chopped (not de-seeded)
- ½ cup extra-virgin olive oil
- 2 tablespoons cider vinegar
- 1 teaspoon honey
- 1 teaspoon sea salt

Instructions

1. Preheat the oven to 150°C regular bake.

Spice Paste:

2. Blitz all the ingredients except the lamb in a food processor to a smooth paste.
3. Spread the spice paste all over the flesh of the lamb, avoiding the fat on top and pushing it into all the nooks and crannies. Cover in plastic wrap and chill for 6 hours, or up to overnight.

To Cook:

1. Scatter the onions over the base of a deep roasting tray that will hold the lamb snugly. Pour in 2 cups of water, then place the lamb on top, skin side up. Sprinkle with sea salt. Cover tightly with foil to seal, then bake for 4 hours.
2. Increase the heat to 180°C regular bake.
3. Uncover the lamb, sprinkle with the cumin seeds and bake for a further 45 minutes, until meltingly tender.

Green Chilli Relsh:

1. Blitz all the ingredients in a small food processor.

To Serve:

2. Carefully transfer the lamb to a serving plate and spoon over some of the cooking juices. Serve with the Green Chilli Relish.

Prep Time: 35 Minutes

Cook Time: 1hrs 30 Minutes

Servings: 4-6

Ingredients

- 6 chicken drumsticks
- 4-5 bone-in, skin-on chicken thighs
- sea salt and ground pepper
- 2 tablespoons olive oil
- 2 brown onions, peeled, cut into quarters through the root
- 2 tablespoons honey
- 2 tablespoons tomato paste
- zest and juice 1 lemon
- 3 tablespoons purchased Moroccan spice mix (I use Simon Gault's)
- 3 cloves garlic, crushed
- 1½ cups pearl couscous (also called mograbieh)
- 3¾ cups chicken stock
- 3 bay leaves
- 1 cinnamon stick

- 12 green or black olives

To serve:

- 2 tablespoons finely chopped pistachios
- 2 tablespoons finely chopped parsley
- Equipment: Large roasting dish or ovenproof baking dish big enough to take everything in a single layer (my tray is 42cm x 32cm x 3cm deep).

Instructions

1. Preheat the oven to 180°C fan bake.
2. Season the chicken with salt and pepper. Heat the oil in a large frying pan and cook the chicken skin side down until deeply golden brown. Transfer to the roasting dish. Don't wash the pan.
3. Add the onions to the pan and cook for 5 minutes, then add to the chicken. In a small bowl, stir the honey, tomato paste, lemon zest and juice, spice mix and garlic together, then tip into the pan and cook for 2 minutes. Stir in

the couscous, stock, bay leaves and the cinnamon stick and bring to the boil.

4. Tip the mixture over the chicken and onions then distribute the couscous evenly so it's not all clumped together and flick off any that's on top of the chicken.

5. Cover tightly with foil and bake for 25 minutes. Uncover, scatter over the olives, then bake for a further 15 minutes, or until the chicken is fully cooked and the couscous is tender but still with a little bite. Scatter over the combined pistachios and parsley.

Prep Time: 35 Minutes

Cook Time: 1hrs 10 Minutes

Servings: 6-8

Ingredients

- 2 Kilograms Beef Cheeks
- 2 Tablespoons Olive Oil
- 80 Grams Pancetta, Chopped
- 1 Onion, Finely Chopped
- 6 Cloves Garlic, Crushed
- 1 Tablespoon Finely Chopped Fresh Rosemary
- 2 Tablespoons Finely Chopped Fresh Oregano
- 2 Tablespoons Tomato Paste
- 2½ Cups Red Wine
- 1 Cup Passata
- 2 Teaspoons Caster Sugar
- Sea Salt And Ground Pepper
- 1 Cup Sunblush Tomatoes, Roughly Chopped
- 16 Large Black Olives

To Serve:

- Hot, Cooked Pappardelle
- Salsa Verde (See Recipe Below)
- 1 Cup Freshly Grated Parmesan

Instructions

1. Trim any sinew from the beef cheeks and cut them in half. Heat the oil in a large casserole dish and, in batches, sear the beef for a few minutes on all sides. Remove from the pan and set aside. Don't wash the pan.

2. Add the pancetta to the pan and cook over a medium-high heat for 3-4 minutes, then reduce the heat and add the onion, garlic, rosemary and oregano. Cook for 10 minutes, until the onion is softened but not coloured. Add the tomato paste, wine, passata and sugar and stir to combine. Season to taste and bring to the boil.

3. Add the beef cheeks back to the pan and bring to the boil. Reduce the heat to low, cover and cook on the stovetop for 3 hours. Stir in the tomatoes and olives and cook for a further 1

hour. Remove and shred the beef cheeks, then add them back to the sauce.

4. To Serve: Serve over hot pappardelle and top with a spoonful of Salsa Verde and parmesan.

5. Cook's note: You can sub out the beef cheeks for stewing steak such as cross-cut, cut into 4cm pieces.

Salsa Verde:

Ingredients

1/3 packed cup each parsley and mint leaves, finely chopped

2 tablespoons capers, roughly chopped

2 cloves garlic, crushed

1 tablespoon lemon juice

pinch caster sugar

3 tablespoons olive oil

sea salt and ground pepper

Method

Combine all the ingredients in a bowl and season with salt and pepper.

DINNERS

21. Simplest Chicken Greek Salad

Prep Time: 15 Minutes

Cook Time: 55 Minutes

Servings: 4

Ingredients

- 2 cups shredded or chopped cooked chicken
- 1 large cucumber, peeled, seeded, and chopped
- 1 red bell pepper, chopped
- 4 Roma tomatoes, chopped
- 1 red onion, chopped
- 1/2 (14–16oz) can garbanzo beans, drained
- 3/4 cup crumbled feta
- 2 Tbsp red wine vinegar
- 1 tsp dried oregano
- Salt and black pepper to taste
- 1/4 cup olive oil

Instructions

1. Combine the chicken, cucumber, bell pepper, tomato, onion, beans, and feta in a large salad bowl.
2. In a separate bowl, combine the vinegar and oregano with a few generous pinches of salt and pepper.
3. Slowly drizzle in the olive oil, whisking to combine.
4. Toss the dressing with the salad.
5. You can serve now, but it's best to let this one sit in the fridge for 30 minutes or so, which gives all the ingredients a chance to get friendly.

Prep Time: 25 Minutes

Cook Time: 55 Minutes

Servings: 6

Ingredients

- ½ Tbsp canola oil
- 1 large onion, sliced
- 1 red bell pepper, sliced
- 1 poblano or green bell pepper, sliced
- Salt and black pepper to taste
- ½ can (14–16oz) black beans, drained
- ¼ tsp cumin
- Juice of 1 lime
- Hot sauce
- 4 (10") whole-wheat tortillas
- cup low-fat shredded Jack cheese
- cups shredded chicken (about half a store-bought rotisserie chicken)
- Salsa (salsa verde is especially good here)

Instructions

1. Heat the oil in a large skillet over high heat.

2. Add the onion and red and poblano peppers and cook until browned, about 7 to 8 minutes. Season with salt and pepper.

3. Combine the beans with cumin in a saucepan and warm through. Add the lime juice and a few shakes of hot sauce.

4. Preheat a griddle, cast-iron skillet, or large nonstick pan over medium heat.

5. Microwave the tortillas for 20 seconds, just enough so they're pliable.

6. Building one burrito at a time, sprinkle on some cheese, top with some beans, the onion-pepper mixture, chicken, and salsa.

7. Roll into a tight package.

8. Place the burritos directly on the skillet, cooking for a minute on each side until lightly toasted.

Prep Time: 25 Minutes

Cook Time: 55 Minutes

Servings: 8

Ingredients

- 1 Tbsp olive oil
- 3 lb ground beef
- 1 medium white onion, chopped
- 1 tsp garlic powder
- 1 tsp onion powder
- 1 tsp kosher salt
- Freshly ground black pepper
- 1/4 cup tomato paste
- 1/4 cup Rao's Marinara Sauce
- 1 1/2 cups heavy cream
- 1 1/4 cup shredded Colby jack cheese
- 1/4 cup chopped chives

Instructions

1. Preheat oven to 375°F.

2. In a very large, shallow pan, heat the oil and add the ground beef. Use a metal pancake turner to press the beef down into a single layer that covers the entire surface of the pan. Cook for 5 to 7 minutes until browned, then use the pancake turner to flip the beef over and cook for another few minutes. Use a large spoon to spoon out excess liquid, until only a small amount remains.

3. Add onion, garlic powder, onion powder, salt, pepper, and tomato paste to the beef. Stir and cook for 1 minute. Add marinara sauce and heavy cream and remove from heat.

4. Stir in 1 cup of shredded cheese and spoon the beef mix into a large casserole dish.

5. Top with remaining cheese and bake about 10 minutes until the cheese is bubbling and melty. Top with chives and serve immediately.

Prep Time: 15 Minutes

Cook Time: 50 Minutes

Servings: 6

Ingredients

- ½ cup reduced-sodium chicken broth
- ¼ cup freshly squeezed lime juice
- 2 Tbsp coconut aminos
- 1 tsp no-sugar-added fish sauce (such as Red Boat)
- 1 tsp honey
- 1 Tbsp coconut oil
- ¼ tsp salt
- ¼ tsp pepper
- 1 medium red onion, halved and thinly sliced
- 2 cloves garlic, minced
- 1 tsp minced fresh ginger
- 1 Thai chili pepper, seeded and very thinly sliced
- 1 pound flank steak, thinly sliced (Note: To make thinner slices, place steak in the freezer for 30 minutes before slicing.)
- 1 (8-ounce) package fresh matchstick-cut carrots

- 2 stalks celery, sliced on the bias
- ½ cup fresh basil leaves, coarsely chopped
- ½ cup fresh mint, coarsely chopped
- 1 (12-ounce) package cauliflower rice, prepared according to package directions

Instructions

1. In a small bowl, stir together broth, lime juice, coconut aminos, fish sauce, and honey; set aside.
2. Heat coconut oil in a large skillet over medium-high heat. Add onion and cook until tender. Add garlic, ginger, and chili pepper; cook 30 seconds or until fragrant. Add meat and sprinkle with salt and black pepper. Cook about 8 minutes or until browned, stirring occasionally. Remove meat mixture from skillet.
3. Add carrot and celery to skillet. Sauté until almost crisp-tender, about 2 minutes. Return meat mixture and accumulated juices to skillet. Add broth mixture and cook and stir until simmering and heated through.
4. Remove skillet from heat. Stir in basil and mint. Serve over cauliflower rice.

Prep Time: 30 Minutes

Cook Time: 55 Minutes

Servings: 6

Ingredients

- 1 lb ground beef
- 2 medium eggs or 1 extra-large egg
- 1/4 cup bread crumbs
- 1/2 cup finely grated Parmesan cheese
- Salt and ground black pepper to taste
- 1/2 Tbsp olive oil
- 1 onion, chopped
- 2 carrots, peeled and chopped
- 2 ribs celery, chopped
- 8 cups low-sodium chicken stock
- 1 head escarole, chopped into bite-size pieces
- 3/4 cup small pasta, like orzo, pastina, or spaghetti broken into 1/2-inch pieces

Instructions

1. Combine the beef with the eggs, bread crumbs, cheese, and good-size pinches of salt and pepper in a mixing bowl.
2. Being careful not to overwork the mixture, lightly form it into meatballs roughly 3/4-inch in diameter, a bit smaller than a golf ball.
3. Heat the olive oil in a large pot over medium-high heat.
4. Add the onion, carrots, and celery and sauté until the vegetables have softened, about 5 minutes.
5. Add the stock and the escarole and bring the soup to a simmer.
6. Turn the heat down to low and add the meatballs and pasta.
7. Simmer for another 8 to 10 minutes, until the meatballs are cooked through and the pasta is al dente.
8. Taste and adjust the seasoning with salt and pepper.
9. Serve the soup with extra cheese on top.

Prep Time: 20 Minutes

Cook Time: 55 Minutes

Servings: 4

Ingredients

- 1Tbsp peanut or vegetable oil
- 4scallions, greens and whites separated, chopped (Scallion greens are best used for garnish at the end, whereas the whites should be used like onions, to build flavor from the beginning.)
- 1Tbsp grated fresh ginger
- 2cloves garlic, minced
- 1medium zucchini, diced
- 2carrots, diced
- 2cups bite-size broccoli florets
- 2cups mushrooms (preferably shiitake), stems removed, sliced
- 1/2 lb boneless, skinless chicken thighs, sliced into thin bite-size pieces
- 4cups cooked brown rice

- 2Tbsp low-sodium soy sauce
- 2eggs, lightly beaten

Instructions

1. In a wok or a large nonstick skillet, heat the oil over medium-high heat.
2. When the oil is lightly smoking, add the scallion whites, ginger, and garlic, and cook for 30 to 45 seconds.
3. Add the zucchini, carrots, broccoli, and mushrooms, and cook for 4 to 5 minutes, using a spatula to stir the vegetables throughout.
4. Add the chicken and continue cooking for 2 to 3 minutes, until the pieces are no longer pink.
5. Stir in the rice and soy sauce, and cook for another 5 minutes, allowing the rice to get crispy on the bottom.
6. Create an empty space in the middle of the pan and add the eggs.
7. Use a spoon or the spatula to quickly scramble the eggs until light and fluffy, then stir them into the rest of the ingredients.
8. Serve garnished with the scallion greens.
9. You might not find it at your local Chinese joint, but really well-made fried rice contains grains with a

lightly crisp, caramelized exterior, which deepens the flavor and the texture of the dish immensely.

10. To achieve that coveted crisp, you'll need to turn up the heat to high during the final moments of cooking. Don't stir the pan—just let the rice sit there for up to 2 minutes as the heat of the pan does its magic.

Prep Time: 20 Minutes

Cook Time: 55 Minutes

Servings: 4

Ingredients

- Prep Time: 1 3 tablespoon canola oil
- 1 teaspoon Chinese five-spice powder
- 4 5-ounce skinless, boneless chicken breast halves
- 4 heads baby bok choy (about 1 lb. total)
- 2 red bell peppers, halved and seeded
- 8 green onions, trimmed
- 2 tablespoon rice vinegar
- 1/4 teaspoon salt
- 1/4 teaspoon black pepper
- 1 cup slivered snow pea pods
- Sesame seeds (optional)

Instructions

1. In a small bowl stir together 1 Tbsp. of the oil and the five-spice powder.

2. Brush chicken, bok choy, peppers, and onions with oil mixture.

3. Use a grill plan to grill chicken and bell peppers, covered, over medium about 10 minutes or until chicken is done (165 °F) and peppers are charred, turning once. Grill bok choy and onions 2 to 4 minutes or until slightly charred, turning once.

4. Transfer chicken and vegetables to a cutting board. Cover chicken to keep warm. Cut vegetables into bite-size pieces.

5. For slaw, in a bowl whisk together the remaining 2 Tbsp. canola oil, the vinegar, salt, and black pepper. Add grilled vegetables and snow pea pods. Toss to combine. Serve chicken with slaw. If desired, sprinkle with sesame seeds.

6. 0 Minutes

Prep Time: 20 Minutes

Cook Time: 55 Minutes

Servings: 4

Ingredients

- 1 Tbsp butter
- 1 yellow onion, diced
- 1 large carrot, diced
- head broccoli, cut into florets and stem thinly sliced
- cloves garlic, chopped
- 1 Tbsp flour
- 1 cup low-sodium chicken stock
- 1 cup beer
- cups milk
- 1 cup shredded sharp Cheddar cheese
- Salt and black pepper to taste
- Tabasco sauce to taste
- Parmesan crisps

Instructions

1. Heat the butter in a large pot over medium heat.
2. Add the onion, carrot, broccoli, and garlic and cook for about 5 minutes, until the vegetables soften.
3. Stir in the flour and cook until it evenly coats all of the vegetables.
4. Add the stock and beer, stirring vigorously to keep the flour from clumping.
5. Simmer for a few minutes, then pour the mixture (working in batches, if need be) into a blender and puree until mostly smooth (a bit of texture can be nice here).
6. You can also use a hand blender to puree the soup in the pot.
7. Return the soup to the pot and bring to a simmer over low heat.
8. Stir in the milk and cheese.
9. After the cheese has fully melted into the soup, season with salt and pepper and a few good shakes of Tabasco.
10. Serve each bowl of soup with a Parmesan crisp floating in the middle.

Prep Time: 30 Minutes

Cook Time: 50 Minutes

Servings: 4-6

Ingredients

- kilogram diced venison
- sea salt and ground pepper
- tablespoons olive oil
- brown onions, thinly sliced
- 2 bay leaves
- cloves garlic, crushed
- 2 teaspoons each dried oregano, ground cumin and smoked paprika
- ½ teaspoon ground cinnamon
- sea salt and ground pepper
- 1 tablespoon each sherry vinegar or red wine vinegar and brown sugar
- 2 whole chipotle peppers in adobo sauce, roughly chopped
- 2 tablespoons each tomato paste, wholegrain mustard, adobo sauce from the peppers and plain flour

- ½ cup red wine

- ¾ cup good-quality beef stock

Crispy Garlicky Crumbs:

- 3 tablespoons olive oil

- tablespoon butter

- 1½ cups fresh sourdough breadcrumbs

- cloves garlic, crushed

- tablespoons finely

- chopped parsley

Instructions

1. Preheat the oven to 120°C regular bake.

2. Trim any silverskin off the venison and season with salt and pepper. Set aside.

3. Heat the oil in an ovenproof casserole dish and add the onions, bay leaves, garlic, oregano and spices with a splash of water. Add a good pinch of salt, cover and cook for 10 minutes over a medium-low heat, stirring often and adding a splash more water if needed. (The water will evaporate off.) Combine the vinegar, sugar, chipotle peppers, tomato paste, mustard, adobo sauce and flour in a bowl, then stir in the wine. Add to the

onions and cook for 3 minutes. Add the stock, season and bring to the boil. Add the seasoned venison to the pot, stir to combine and heat until it just comes to the boil. Press a circle of baking paper down onto the meat then cover the dish tightly with a lid or foil. Place in the oven and cook for 50 minutes, stirring after 30 minutes.

Crumbs:

1. Heat the oil and butter in a large frying pan and cook the crumbs until golden and crisp, stirring often. Stir in the garlic and parsley and season well. Scatter over the venison when serving.
2. Cook's note: We served the venison with mashed potatoes and flash-fried green beans.

Prep Time: 30 Minutes

Cook Time: 50 Minutes

Servings: 2

Ingredients

Sauce:

- 3 tablespoons gochujang (Korean red pepper paste)
- 2 tablespoons honey
- tablespoon soy sauce
- 1 tablespoon grated fresh ginger
- cloves garlic, crushed
- teaspoons sesame oil
- 2 teaspoons rice vinegar
- ½-1 teaspoon chilli flakes, to taste

To cook and serve:

- 300 grams beef schnitzel, sliced into very thin strips (see Cook's note)
- sea salt and ground pepper
- vegetable oil

- 200 grams slim green beans, thinly sliced on the diagonal
- 1½ cups kimchi
- toasted sesame seeds and finely chopped coriander, to serve
- hot cooked noodles or rice, to serve

Instructions

1. Sauce: Mix all the ingredients together and set aside.
2. To cook and serve: Season the steak with salt and pepper. Heats a large frying pan with a little oil until searing hot. Add the steak in small batches and cook for 10-15 seconds. Transfer to a plate and cover to keep warm while you cook the remaining steak. Add a little more oil to the pan, add the beans and cook until lightly blistered. Add the kimchi and cook for 2 minutes, tossing together. Tip in the sauce and let it bubble up. Add the beef and resting juices and stir everything together.
3. Divide between bowls and top with the sesame seeds and coriander. Serve with noodles or rice.
4. Cook's note: The steak needs to be wafer-thin so it will cook in seconds and remain tender. Place the

schnitzel between 2 pieces of plastic wrap and flatten with a rolling pin before cutting into 2cm-wide strips.

www.ingramcontent.com/pod-product-compliance
Lightning Source LLC
Chambersburg PA
CBHW061516250726
48657CB00005B/1904